ULCERATIVE COLITIS DIET COOKBOOK FOR BEGINNERS

NATALIE BROWN

Copyright ©2023.

This work is protected by copyright law. All rights reserved. No part of this book may be reproduced, stored in a retrieval system, transmitted in any form or by any means, electronic, mechanical, photocopying, recording, or otherwise, without the prior written consent of the copyright holder. The unauthorized reproduction, distribution, or creation of derivative works of this work is strictly prohibited and may be punishable under copyright law. The copyright holder reserves the right to pursue any and all legal remedies against any person or entity that violates the rights granted by copyright law.

TABLE OF CONTENTS

UNDERSTANDING ULCERATIVE COLITIS...3

FOOD TO EAT AND FOOD TO AVOID............8

BENEFITS OF FOLLOWING ULCERATIVE COLITIS DIET 14

HOW TO A FOLLOW A UC DIET...................18

SHOPPING INGREDIENTS LIST FOR UC DIET 22

COMPLICATIONS OF A UC DISEASE DIET.25

MEAL PLANNING..................29

21-DAY MEAL PLAN FOR A UC DIET..........33

UC DIET BREAKFAST RECIPES....................44

UC DIET LUNCH RECIPES 64

UC DIET DINNER RECIPES 84

CONCLUSION 107

UNDERSTANDING ULCERATIVE COLITIS

Ulcerative colitis is a chronic inflammatory bowel disease (IBD) that primarily affects the colon and rectum. It is characterized by inflammation and ulcers in the inner lining of the colon, leading to a range of symptoms and potential complications. Understanding the types, causes, symptoms, and preventive measures of ulcerative colitis is crucial for managing and minimizing its impact on individuals' lives.

TYPES OF ULCERATIVE COLITIS:

There are several types of ulcerative colitis based on the extent of inflammation in the colon:

1. **Ulcerative Proctitis:** Inflammation is limited to the rectum.
2. **Proctosigmoiditis:** Inflammation extends into the sigmoid colon.

3. **Left-sided Colitis:** Inflammation reaches up to the descending colon.
4. **Pancolitis:** Inflammation affects the entire colon.

CAUSES OF ULCERATIVE COLITIS:

The exact cause of ulcerative colitis is not fully understood, but it is believed to result from a combination of genetic, environmental, and immune system factors. A genetic predisposition plays a role, as individuals with a family history of IBD are at a higher risk. Environmental triggers, such as diet, stress, and certain infections, might also contribute. The immune system's response to these triggers leads to chronic inflammation in the colon.

SYMPTOMS OF ULCERATIVE COLITIS:

The symptoms of ulcerative colitis can vary in intensity and may include:

- **Abdominal pain:** Cramping and discomfort are common due to inflammation.

- **Diarrhea:** Frequent and urgent bowel movements often containing blood or mucus.
- **Rectal bleeding:** Blood in stools due to ulcers in the colon lining.
- **Weight loss:** Chronic inflammation can affect nutrient absorption.
- **Fatigue:** Inflammation and other symptoms can lead to reduced energy levels.
- **Fever:** In severe cases, fever might indicate infection or inflammation.
- **Anemia:** Chronic bleeding can lead to a decrease in red blood cell count.
- **Joint pain:** Inflammation might extend to joints, causing pain.
- **Skin issues:** Some individuals experience skin problems like rashes.

PREVENTIVE MEASURES:

While there is no known cure for ulcerative colitis, certain preventive measures can help manage symptoms and reduce the risk of flare-ups:

1. **Medication Compliance:** Adhering to prescribed medications, such as anti-inflammatory drugs and immune system modulators, can help control inflammation and maintain remission.
2. **Dietary Changes:** Identifying trigger foods and maintaining a balanced diet can alleviate symptoms. Some individuals find relief by avoiding spicy, fatty, or high-fiber foods during flare-ups.
3. **Stress Management:** Stress can exacerbate symptoms. Techniques like meditation, yoga, and deep breathing can help manage stress and potentially reduce flare-ups.
4. **Hydration**: Staying hydrated supports overall gastrointestinal health and can ease some symptoms.
5. **Regular Exercise:** Physical activity can help improve digestion, manage stress, and maintain overall well-being.
6. **Consulting a Specialist:** Regular check-ups with a gastroenterologist are essential to

monitor the condition and adjust the treatment plan as needed.
7. **Avoiding Smoking:** Smoking can worsen symptoms and increase the risk of complications. Quitting smoking is recommended.
8. **Informed Lifestyle Choices:** Educating oneself about ulcerative colitis and seeking support from patient communities can provide valuable insights and emotional support.

FOOD TO EAT AND FOOD TO AVOID

Creating a suitable diet for ulcerative colitis (UC) is crucial in managing symptoms and promoting overall health. While dietary needs can vary from person to person, there are certain foods that individuals with UC should generally consider avoiding to achieve optimum health:

FOOD TO EAT

- **Low-Fiber Foods:** Opt for cooked, peeled, and well-cooked fruits and vegetables. Examples include bananas, applesauce, cooked carrots, squash, and potatoes. These options are gentler on the digestive system and less likely to cause irritation.
- **Lean Proteins:** Incorporate lean protein sources such as skinless poultry, fish, eggs, and tofu. These provide essential amino

acids without adding unnecessary strain on digestion.
- **Cooked Grains:** Choose refined grains like white rice, refined pasta, and oatmeal. These are easier to digest compared to whole grains and provide a good source of energy.
- **Dairy Alternatives:** If dairy is problematic, opt for lactose-free dairy products or plant-based alternatives like almond milk, coconut milk, or lactose-free yogurt.
- **Healthy Fats:** Include sources of healthy fats like avocados, olive oil, and nuts. These fats can provide a good source of energy and support overall health.
- **Cooked Fruits:** Cooked or stewed fruits like apples or pears can be easier to digest than raw ones. These can also provide important vitamins and minerals.
- **Well-Cooked Vegetables:** Steamed or boiled vegetables such as spinach, zucchini, and green beans can be more easily tolerated. Be sure to cook them until they are soft to minimize digestive strain.

- **Nut Butters:** Smooth nut butters like peanut butter or almond butter can provide protein and healthy fats without the added fiber found in whole nuts.
- **Probiotic Foods:** Incorporating probiotic-rich foods like yogurt or fermented foods (kimchi, sauerkraut, kefir) can help promote a healthy gut microbiome.
- **Hydration:** Staying hydrated is crucial. Drink water, herbal teas, and clear broths to prevent dehydration, which can worsen symptoms.
- **Small, Frequent Meals:** Consuming smaller, more frequent meals can help ease the burden on your digestive system and prevent overloading it.
- **Well-Cooked Meats:** Lean meats that are well-cooked and tender can provide protein without being hard to digest.
- **Eggs**: Eggs are a versatile and easily digestible protein source that can be prepared in various ways.

- **Smoothies:** Blending easily digestible ingredients like yogurt, ripe bananas, and cooked fruits can create a nutrient-rich and soothing option.

FOOD TO AVOID

1. High-Fiber Foods: Foods rich in insoluble fiber, such as whole grains, nuts, seeds, and raw vegetables, can exacerbate digestive symptoms in individuals with UC. These foods can be hard to digest and might contribute to diarrhea and abdominal discomfort. Opt for well-cooked and peeled fruits and vegetables, and consider low-fiber alternatives like white rice and refined pasta.

2. Spicy Foods: Spices and spicy foods can trigger inflammation and irritation in the digestive tract, leading to discomfort for those with UC. It's advisable to avoid or limit foods seasoned with hot spices, chili, or excessive amounts of pepper.

3. Dairy Products: Dairy products can be problematic for individuals with UC, especially during flare-ups. Lactose intolerance might worsen symptoms. Opt for lactose-free dairy alternatives like almond milk or lactose-free yogurt. However, some individuals with UC might tolerate dairy well, so it's important to gauge your personal response.

4. Caffeine and Carbonated Drinks: Caffeine and carbonation can stimulate the digestive system and potentially cause irritation. Coffee, tea, soda, and energy drinks should be consumed in moderation or avoided, especially during flare-ups.

5. Fatty and Fried Foods: High-fat and fried foods can be difficult to digest and may trigger inflammation. Foods like fried chicken, French fries, and fatty cuts of meat should be limited. Opt for lean protein sources and healthier cooking methods like baking, grilling, or steaming.

6. Artificial Sweeteners: Artificial sweeteners like sorbitol and mannitol, commonly found in sugar-free gum, candies, and some diet beverages, can have a laxative effect and worsen diarrhea.

7. Alcohol: Alcohol can irritate the digestive tract and contribute to dehydration. It's best to avoid or limit alcohol consumption, especially during active flare-ups.

8. Raw Vegetables and Fruits with Skin: The skin of certain fruits and vegetables can be tough to digest and may contribute to discomfort. Peeling and cooking fruits and vegetables can make them easier on the digestive system.

9. High-Sugar Foods: Sugary foods and beverages can cause rapid fluctuations in blood sugar levels and potentially worsen inflammation. Reducing the consumption of sugary snacks, candies, and sweetened beverages is advisable.

10. Processed Foods: Processed foods often contain additives, preservatives, and unhealthy fats that might trigger inflammation and exacerbate UC symptoms. Opt for whole, natural foods whenever possible.

BENEFITS OF FOLLOWING ULCERATIVE COLITIS DIET

Following an ulcerative colitis (UC) disease diet can have a range of core benefits, especially for beginners who are just starting to navigate the dietary adjustments necessary to manage their condition. Here are the key advantages of adopting a UC-specific diet:

1. Symptom Management: A tailored UC diet can help reduce the frequency and severity of symptoms such as abdominal pain, diarrhea, and rectal bleeding. By avoiding trigger foods, individuals can experience fewer flare-ups and improved comfort.

2. Inflammation Reduction: A well-chosen UC diet can contribute to decreasing inflammation in the digestive tract. This is vital, as chronic inflammation is a hallmark of the disease and is responsible for many of its symptoms and complications.

3. Improved Nutrient Absorption: UC can sometimes lead to malabsorption of nutrients due to inflammation in the intestines. A carefully designed diet can ensure that the body is getting the necessary vitamins, minerals, and nutrients to maintain overall health.

4. Weight Management: UC can cause unintended weight loss or gain. A balanced UC diet can help maintain a healthy weight by providing the body with the appropriate nutrients and energy it needs.

5. Enhanced Gut Health: Certain foods in a UC diet, such as probiotic-rich options like yogurt or fermented foods, can support the growth of beneficial gut bacteria. A healthier gut microbiome may positively impact digestion and overall well-being.

6. Prevention of Nutrient Deficiencies: Chronic inflammation and frequent bowel movements can lead to nutrient deficiencies. A well-structured UC diet can help prevent deficiencies in important nutrients like iron, calcium, vitamin D, and B vitamins.

7. Increased Energy Levels: By avoiding trigger foods and incorporating nourishing options, individuals can experience increased energy levels, improved concentration, and better overall vitality.

8. Reduction in Bowel Discomfort: Following a UC diet can lead to a decrease in bowel discomfort, including cramping, gas, and bloating. This can greatly improve quality of life.

9. Psychological Well-being: Managing UC symptoms can be emotionally challenging. A diet that helps control symptoms can lead to improved mental health and a better sense of control over the condition.

10. Personalized Approach: Every individual's response to different foods can vary. A UC diet is not a one-size-fits-all approach. It's tailored to the individual's needs, preferences, and sensitivities, ensuring a more personalized and effective approach.

11. Reduced Dependency on Medication: While medication is often necessary, an appropriate UC diet can potentially lead to reduced dependency on certain medications, improving the individual's overall health.

12. Long-Term Disease Management: By adopting a UC diet from the beginning, individuals can establish healthy eating habits that will contribute to long-term disease management and a higher quality of life.

13. Supportive Lifestyle: Following a UC diet often goes hand-in-hand with other healthy lifestyle habits, such as managing stress, staying hydrated, and engaging in regular physical activity. These habits collectively contribute to a healthier and more balanced lifestyle.

14. Empowerment: Learning about foods that support your health and those that can trigger symptoms empowers you to take an active role in managing your condition. This knowledge can boost confidence and reduce anxiety surrounding meal choices.

HOW TO A FOLLOW A UC DIET

Following an ulcerative colitis (UC) disease diet requires careful planning and dedication. Here's a step-by-step guide on how to effectively follow a UC-specific diet:

1. **Consult a Healthcare Professional:** Before making any significant dietary changes, consult a gastroenterologist or a registered dietitian with expertise in gastrointestinal health. They can provide personalized guidance based on your specific condition, needs, and goals.
2. **Understand Trigger Foods:** Learn about foods that commonly trigger UC symptoms. These can vary from person to person, but common triggers include high-fiber foods, spicy foods, dairy, caffeine, and fatty foods.
3. **Keep a Food Journal**: Start a food journal to track your meals, snacks, symptoms, and

how your body responds to different foods. This can help identify patterns and specific trigger foods.
4. **Create a Meal Plan:** Work with a dietitian to create a meal plan that includes a variety of nutrient-rich, easily digestible foods. Plan balanced meals and snacks that cater to your dietary restrictions and preferences.
5. **Gradual Changes:** Transition to your new diet gradually. Sudden dietary shifts can cause digestive discomfort. Slowly introduce new foods and monitor your body's response.
6. **Focus on Low-Fiber Options:** Especially during flare-ups, opt for low-fiber foods like well-cooked vegetables, cooked fruits, white rice, and refined grains.
7. **Include Lean Proteins:** Incorporate lean protein sources such as skinless poultry, fish, eggs, and tofu. These are typically easier to digest.
8. **Monitor Lactose Intolerance:** If you're lactose intolerant, consider avoiding or

limiting dairy products. Opt for lactose-free alternatives or dairy-free options.
9. **Experiment with Probiotics:** Some individuals find that probiotic-rich foods or supplements support their gut health. Experiment with these under the guidance of a healthcare professional.
10. **Stay Hydrated:** Drink plenty of water throughout the day to prevent dehydration, which can worsen UC symptoms.
11. **Avoid Processed Foods:** Limit or avoid highly processed foods that often contain additives, preservatives, and unhealthy fats.
12. **Learn Portion Control:** Pay attention to portion sizes. Eating smaller, more frequent meals can be easier on your digestive system.
13. **Manage Stress:** Stress can trigger UC flare-ups. Practice stress-reducing techniques like meditation, deep breathing, and gentle exercise.
14. **Plan Snacks:** Have UC-friendly snacks on hand to avoid reaching for trigger foods

when hungry. Consider options like rice cakes, plain yogurt, and nut butter.
15. **Monitor Symptoms:** Continuously monitor your symptoms and how your body reacts to different foods. Adjust your diet based on your observations.
16. **Reintroduce Foods:** As you gain control over your symptoms, gradually reintroduce foods you previously avoided. Do this one at a time to identify how your body responds.
17. **Be Patient**: Finding the right diet that works for you might take time. Stay patient, and don't get discouraged by setbacks.
18. **Regular Follow-ups:** Regularly meet with your healthcare professional or dietitian to discuss your progress, make adjustments to your diet plan, and address any concerns.

SHOPPING INGREDIENTS LIST FOR UC DIET

Here's a list of healthy shopping ingredients that can be beneficial for an ulcerative colitis disease diet. These items are generally well-tolerated and can help support your digestive health:

- **White Rice:** An easily digestible source of carbohydrates that can be used as a base for meals.
- **Oatmeal:** Provides soluble fiber that can help regulate digestion and promote a feeling of fullness.
- **Skinless Poultry:** Lean protein from chicken or turkey is often well-tolerated and provides essential amino acids.
- **Fish:** Fatty fish like salmon, mackerel, and trout are rich in omega-3 fatty acids, which have anti-inflammatory properties.

- **Eggs:** A versatile source of protein that can be prepared in various ways.
- **Tofu:** A plant-based protein option that is easy to digest and can be used in various dishes.
- **Cooked Carrots:** A gentle vegetable that provides vitamins and minerals without excessive fiber.
- **Cooked Spinach:** A nutrient-rich green that can be cooked until soft for easier digestion.
- **Ripe Bananas:** A soft and easily digestible fruit that can provide energy and important nutrients.
- **Applesauce:** Provides the benefits of apples without the skin, making it easier on the digestive system.
- **Almond Milk:** A dairy-free alternative that can be used in smoothies, cereal, or cooking.
- **Nut Butters:** Smooth nut butters like peanut or almond butter offer healthy fats and protein.

- **Low-Fat Yogurt:** If tolerated, yogurt with live cultures can contribute to a healthier gut microbiome.
- **Lactose-Free Dairy:** Consider lactose-free milk and yogurt options if you are sensitive to lactose.
- **White Bread or Rolls:** Choose refined grains for baked goods to minimize fiber content.
- **Low-Fiber Pasta:** Opt for pasta made from refined grains for a more easily digestible option.
- **Ripe Avocado:** A source of healthy fats that can be added to smoothies or used as a spread.
- **Cooked Zucchini:** A mild and easily digestible vegetable that can be incorporated into various dishes.
- **Ripe Papaya:** Contains enzymes that can aid digestion and promote gut health.
- **Bone Broth:** A soothing and hydrating option that can help support digestion and provide nutrients.

COMPLICATIONS OF A UC DISEASE DIET

If the right diet isn't adopted for managing ulcerative colitis (UC), several complications can arise due to uncontrolled inflammation and worsening of symptoms. Here are some potential complications:

1. **Flare-Ups:** Without a proper diet, the risk of frequent and severe flare-ups increases. These flare-ups can lead to debilitating symptoms like intense abdominal pain, diarrhea, rectal bleeding, and fatigue.
2. **Malnutrition:** Inadequate nutrient intake due to a poor diet can lead to malnutrition. Chronic inflammation and frequent bowel movements can hinder the absorption of essential nutrients, potentially resulting in weight loss, weakness, and deficiencies in vitamins and minerals.

3. **Dehydration:** Diarrhea and frequent bowel movements can lead to dehydration, especially if fluid intake is not sufficient. Dehydration can worsen symptoms and lead to complications like electrolyte imbalances and kidney issues.
4. **Anemia:** Chronic bleeding and poor nutrient absorption can lead to anemia, a condition characterized by a reduced number of red blood cells. Anemia can cause fatigue, weakness, and other complications.
5. **Intestinal Strictures:** Prolonged inflammation can lead to the development of scar tissue and narrowing of the intestines, known as strictures. This can obstruct the flow of digested food and lead to bowel obstruction.
6. **Perforation:** Severe inflammation can weaken the walls of the colon, increasing the risk of perforation (tearing) of the intestinal lining. This can lead to a life-threatening condition requiring emergency medical intervention.

7. **Toxic Megacolon:** In rare cases, uncontrolled inflammation can cause the colon to enlarge significantly, a condition known as toxic megacolon. This is a medical emergency and requires immediate treatment.
8. **Increased Cancer Risk:** Long-standing inflammation in the colon is associated with an increased risk of developing colon cancer. Adopting a diet that supports gut health and minimizes inflammation is crucial for reducing this risk.
9. **Joint Pain and Inflammation:** Some individuals with UC may experience joint pain and inflammation, a condition known as arthralgia. An improper diet can exacerbate joint symptoms.
10. **Impact on Mental Health:** Living with uncontrolled UC symptoms due to a poor diet can negatively impact mental health, leading to increased stress, anxiety, and depression.

11. **Medication Dependency:** Without dietary support, individuals might become more reliant on medication to manage symptoms, leading to potential side effects and decreased quality of life.
12. **Reduced Quality of Life:** The combination of ongoing symptoms, complications, and lifestyle limitations can significantly reduce overall quality of life for individuals with UC.

MEAL PLANNING

Meal planning is a strategic approach to structuring your meals and snacks in a way that supports the management of ulcerative colitis (UC) symptoms. This involves choosing the right foods, portions, and timing to help minimize inflammation, discomfort, and other complications associated with the condition. Here's how meal planning can benefit the proper management of UC:

1. **Avoiding Trigger Foods:** By planning your meals in advance, you can consciously avoid trigger foods that exacerbate UC symptoms. This prevents unexpected flare-ups and discomfort.
2. **Balancing Nutrient Intake:** Meal planning ensures you receive a balanced intake of essential nutrients like vitamins, minerals, protein, and healthy fats. This supports overall health and helps prevent malnutrition.

3. **Portion Control:** Planning portions helps prevent overeating, which can strain the digestive system. Eating smaller, more frequent meals can reduce the burden on your gut.
4. **Consistency:** Consistent meal timing and choices can help regulate digestion and bowel movements. This predictability can reduce the chances of sudden symptoms.
5. **Stress Reduction:** Planning your meals in advance eliminates the stress of last-minute decisions, making eating a more relaxed and mindful experience. Stress reduction is vital for managing UC.
6. **Hydration:** Incorporating fluids and hydrating foods into your meal plan helps prevent dehydration, a common issue among UC patients due to diarrhea.
7. **Adequate Fiber Intake:** Proper meal planning ensures that you can include fiber-rich foods that are gentle on the digestive system, promoting regular bowel movements without triggering symptoms.

8. **Integration of Gut-Friendly Foods:** Planning meals allows you to incorporate probiotic-rich foods like yogurt or fermented foods, which can support gut health and reduce inflammation.
9. **Reducing Flare-Up Risks:** By avoiding foods that are known to trigger flare-ups and focusing on foods that soothe inflammation, you can significantly reduce the risk of experiencing sudden symptoms.
10. **Supporting Medication Efficacy:** A well-planned diet can complement the effects of medications by providing the necessary nutrients for overall health and healing.
11. **Improved Mental Health:** Following a meal plan can alleviate the stress of decision-making, which is especially important for individuals with UC, as stress can exacerbate symptoms.
12. **Long-Term Management:** Meal planning helps you establish sustainable eating habits, making it easier to manage UC over the long term and reducing the risk of complications.

13. **Confidence and Empowerment:** Knowing what you'll eat in advance gives you a sense of control and confidence in your dietary choices, fostering a positive mindset toward managing your condition.
14. **Easier Social Engagements:** With a meal plan, you can better navigate social situations that involve food, ensuring you make choices that align with your dietary needs.

21-DAY MEAL PLAN FOR A UC DIET

DAY 1:

- **Breakfast**: Scrambled eggs with cooked spinach and white rice.
- **Lunch:** Grilled chicken breast with mashed potatoes and well-cooked carrots.
- **Snack:** Ripe banana with almond butter.
- **Dinner:** Baked salmon with steamed zucchini and white rice.

DAY 2:

- **Breakfast:** Oatmeal cooked with almond milk, topped with ripe papaya and a sprinkle of cinnamon.

- **Lunch:** Tofu stir-fry with bell peppers, broccoli, and a low-fiber pasta.
- **Snack:** Rice cake with a small serving of low-fat yogurt.
- **Dinner:** Turkey meatballs with white rice and cooked green beans.

DAY 3:

- **Breakfast:** Smoothie with ripe banana, lactose-free yogurt, almond milk, and a spoonful of nut butter.
- **Lunch:** Grilled fish tacos with soft tortillas, lettuce, and tomato.
- **Snack:** Cooked applesauce with a sprinkle of cinnamon.
- **Dinner:** Lean beef stew with well-cooked carrots and white rice.

DAY 4:

- **Breakfast:** Greek yogurt with ripe berries and a drizzle of honey.
- **Lunch:** Quinoa salad with cooked chicken, cucumber, and avocado.
- **Snack:** Rice cake with hummus.
- **Dinner:** Baked chicken with mashed potatoes and steamed zucchini.

DAY 5:

- **Breakfast:** Scrambled eggs with cooked spinach and white rice.
- **Lunch:** Vegetable and rice soup with well-cooked vegetables.
- **Snack:** Nut and dried fruit mix.
- **Dinner:** Grilled salmon with quinoa and cooked carrots.

DAY 6:

- **Breakfast**: Oatmeal cooked with almond milk, topped with ripe papaya and a sprinkle of cinnamon.
- **Lunch:** Tofu and vegetable stir-fry with white rice.
- **Snack:** Rice cake with almond butter.
- **Dinner:** Turkey burger with a side of mashed potatoes and cooked green beans.

DAY 7:

- **Breakfast:** Smoothie with ripe banana, lactose-free yogurt, almond milk, and a spoonful of nut butter.
- **Lunch:** Chicken wrap with soft tortilla, lettuce, tomato, and hummus.
- **Snack:** Greek yogurt with ripe berries.
- **Dinner:** Baked fish with quinoa and well-cooked zucchini.

DAY 8:

- **Breakfast:** Smoothie with ripe banana, lactose-free yogurt, almond milk, and a spoonful of nut butter.
- **Lunch:** Turkey meatballs with white rice and cooked green beans.
- **Snack:** Rice cake with hummus.
- **Dinner:** Grilled chicken breast with mashed potatoes and well-cooked carrots.

DAY 9:

- **Breakfast:** Greek yogurt with ripe berries and a drizzle of honey.
- **Lunch:** Baked salmon with steamed zucchini and white rice.
- **Snack:** Ripe banana with almond butter.
- **Dinner:** Tofu stir-fry with bell peppers, broccoli, and a low-fiber pasta.

DAY 10:

- **Breakfast:** Oatmeal cooked with almond milk, topped with ripe papaya and a sprinkle of cinnamon.
- **Lunch:** Quinoa salad with cooked chicken, cucumber, and avocado.
- **Snack:** Nut and dried fruit mix.
- **Dinner:** Lean beef stew with well-cooked carrots and white rice.

DAY 11:

- **Breakfast:** Scrambled eggs with cooked spinach and white rice.
- **Lunch:** Vegetable and rice soup with well-cooked vegetables.
- **Snack:** Cooked applesauce with a sprinkle of cinnamon.
- **Dinner:** Turkey burger with a side of mashed potatoes and cooked green beans.

DAY 12:

- **Breakfast:** Smoothie with ripe banana, lactose-free yogurt, almond milk, and a spoonful of nut butter.

- **Lunch:** Chicken wrap with soft tortilla, lettuce, tomato, and hummus.

- **Snack:** Greek yogurt with ripe berries.

- **Dinner:** Grilled fish tacos with soft tortillas, lettuce, and tomato.

DAY 13:

- **Breakfast:** Oatmeal cooked with almond milk, topped with ripe papaya and a sprinkle of cinnamon.

- **Lunch:** Tofu and vegetable stir-fry with white rice.

- **Snack:** Rice cake with almond butter.

- **Dinner:** Baked chicken with mashed potatoes and steamed zucchini.

DAY 14:

- **Breakfast:** Scrambled eggs with cooked spinach and white rice.
- **Lunch:** Grilled salmon with quinoa and cooked carrots.
- **Snack:** Rice cake with a small serving of low-fat yogurt.
- **Dinner:** Lean beef stew with well-cooked vegetables and white rice.

DAY 15:

- **Breakfast:** Smoothie with ripe banana, lactose-free yogurt, almond milk, and a spoonful of nut butter.
- **Lunch:** Turkey meatballs with white rice and cooked green beans.
- **Snack:** Rice cake with hummus.
- **Dinner:** Grilled chicken breast with mashed potatoes and well-cooked carrots.

DAY 16:

- **Breakfast:** Greek yogurt with ripe berries and a drizzle of honey.
- **Lunch:** Baked salmon with steamed zucchini and white rice.
- **Snack:** Ripe banana with almond butter.
- **Dinner:** Tofu stir-fry with bell peppers, broccoli, and a low-fiber pasta.

DAY 17:

- **Breakfast:** Oatmeal cooked with almond milk, topped with ripe papaya and a sprinkle of cinnamon.
- **Lunch:** Quinoa salad with cooked chicken, cucumber, and avocado.
- **Snack:** Nut and dried fruit mix.
- **Dinner:** Lean beef stew with well-cooked carrots and white rice.

DAY 18:

- **Breakfast:** Scrambled eggs with cooked spinach and white rice.
- **Lunch:** Vegetable and rice soup with well-cooked vegetables.
- **Snack:** Cooked applesauce with a sprinkle of cinnamon.
- **Dinner:** Turkey burger with a side of mashed potatoes and cooked green beans.

DAY 19:

- **Breakfast:** Smoothie with ripe banana, lactose-free yogurt, almond milk, and a spoonful of nut butter.
- **Lunch:** Chicken wrap with soft tortilla, lettuce, tomato, and hummus.
- **Snack:** Greek yogurt with ripe berries.
- **Dinner:** Grilled fish tacos with soft tortillas, lettuce, and tomato.

DAY 20:

- **Breakfast:** Oatmeal cooked with almond milk, topped with ripe papaya and a sprinkle of cinnamon.
- **Lunch:** Tofu and vegetable stir-fry with white rice.
- **Snack:** Rice cake with almond butter.
- **Dinner:** Baked chicken with mashed potatoes and steamed zucchini.

DAY 21:

- **Breakfast:** Scrambled eggs with cooked spinach and white rice.
- **Lunch:** Grilled salmon with quinoa and cooked carrots.
- **Snack:** Rice cake with a small serving of low-fat yogurt.
- **Dinner:** Lean beef stew with well-cooked vegetables and white rice.

UC DIET BREAKFAST RECIPES

1. SCRAMBLED EGGS WITH SPINACH AND RICE:

INGREDIENTS:

- 2 large eggs
- 1 cup fresh spinach, chopped
- 1/2 cup cooked white rice

INSTRUCTION

- In a bowl, whisk the eggs.
- Heat a non-stick skillet over medium heat and add the eggs.
- Once the eggs start to set, add the chopped spinach and continue to scramble until cooked.

- Serve over cooked white rice.

Nutritional Value: Approximately 250 calories, 15g protein, 10g fat, 25g carbohydrates.

Cooking Time: 10 minutes

2. BANANA ALMOND BUTTER SMOOTHIE:

INGREDIENTS:

- 1 ripe banana
- 1 tablespoon almond butter
- 1/2 cup lactose-free yogurt
- 1/2 cup almond milk

INSTRUCTION

1. Blend all the ingredients until smooth.
2. If desired, add ice for a colder texture.

Nutritional Value: Approximately 300 calories, 6g protein, 15g fat, 35g carbohydrates.

Preparation Time: 5 minutes

3. GREEK YOGURT PARFAIT:

INGREDIENTS:

- 1/2 cup lactose-free Greek yogurt
- 1/4 cup ripe berries (blueberries, strawberries, raspberries)
- 2 tablespoons chopped nuts (almonds, walnuts)

INSTRUCTION

1. In a glass, layer yogurt, berries, and chopped nuts.
2. Repeat the layers as desired.

Nutritional Value: Approximately 200 calories, 10g protein, 10g fat, 20g carbohydrates.

Preparation Time: 5 minutes

4. PAPAYA OATMEAL BOWL:

INGREDIENTS:

- 1/2 cup oatmeal
- 1 cup almond milk
- 1/2 ripe papaya, diced
- 1 tablespoon honey (optional)

INSTRUCTION

1. Cook oatmeal in almond milk according to package instructions.
2. Top with diced papaya and drizzle with honey if desired.

Nutritional Value: Approximately 300 calories, 6g protein, 5g fat, 55g carbohydrates.

Cooking Time: 10 minutes

5. RICE CAKE WITH NUT BUTTER AND BANANA:

INGREDIENTS:

- 1 rice cake
- 1tablespoonalmondbutterorpeanut butter
- 1/2 ripe banana, sliced

INSTRUCTION

1. Spread nut butter on the rice cake.
2. Top with sliced banana.

Nutritional Value: Approximately 200 calories, 4g protein, 10g fat, 25g carbohydrates.

Preparation Time: 2 minutes

6. SPINACH AND CHEESE OMELETTE:

INGREDIENTS:

- 2 large eggs
- 1 cup fresh spinach, chopped
- 1/4 cup grated cheddar cheese (lactose-free if needed)

INSTRUCTION

1. In a bowl, whisk the eggs.
2. Heat a non-stick skillet over medium heat and pour in the eggs.
3. Sprinkle chopped spinach and cheese on one half of the omelette.
4. Fold the other half over the filling and cook until set.

Nutritional Value: Approximately 300 calories, 15g protein, 20g fat, 5g carbohydrates.

Cooking Time: 10 minutes

7. RIPE BANANA PANCAKES:

INGREDIENTS:

- 1 ripe banana
- 2 eggs

INSTRUCTION

1. Mash the ripe banana in a bowl.
2. Whisk in the eggs until well combined.
3. Heat a non-stick skillet over medium heat and pour small amounts of the batter to make pancakes.
4. Cook until bubbles form on the surface, then flip and cook until golden.

Nutritional Value: Approximately 250 calories, 10g protein, 10g fat, 30g carbohydrates.

Cooking Time: 15 minutes

8. COOKED APPLESAUCE WITH CINNAMON:

INGREDIENTS:

- 2 apples, peeled, cored, and diced
- 1/2 teaspoon cinnamon

INSTRUCTION

1. In a pot, combine diced apples and a splash of water.
2. Cook over low heat until the apples are soft and easily mashed.
3. Mash the apples with a fork and stir in cinnamon.

Nutritional Value: Approximately 150 calories, 1g protein, 0g fat, 40g carbohydrates.

Cooking Time: 15 minutes

9. QUINOA BREAKFAST BOWL:

INGREDIENTS:

- 1/2 cup cooked quinoa
- 1/4 cup lactose-free Greek yogurt
- 1/4 cup ripe berries
- 1 tablespoon chopped nuts (almonds, walnuts)

INSTRUCTION

1. In a bowl, layer quinoa, Greek yogurt, berries, and chopped nuts.

Nutritional Value: Approximately 250 calories, 8g protein, 10g fat, 30g carbohydrates.

Preparation Time: 5 minutes

10. NUT AND DRIED FRUIT MIX:

INGREDIENTS:

- 1/4 cup mixed nuts (almonds, walnuts, cashews)
- 1/4 cup dried cranberries or raisins

INSTRUCTION

1. Combine mixed nuts and dried cranberries in a bowl.
2. Enjoy as a simple and quick on-the-go breakfast.

Nutritional Value: Approximately 250 calories, 6g protein, 15g fat, 25g carbohydrates.

Preparation Time: 2 minutes

11. AVOCADO RICE CAKE:

INGREDIENTS:

- 1 rice cake
- 1/4 ripe avocado, mashed
- Pinch of salt and pepper

INSTRUCTION

1. Spread mashed avocado on the rice cake.
2. Sprinkle with a pinch of salt and pepper.

Nutritional Value: Approximately 150 calories, 2g protein, 8g fat, 20g carbohydrates.

Preparation Time: 5 minutes

12. BERRY CHIA PUDDING:

INGREDIENTS:

- 2 tablespoons chia seeds
- 1/2 cup almond milk
- 1/4 cup ripe berries

INSTRUCTION

1. In a bowl, combine chia seeds and almond milk. Stir well.
2. Refrigerate for a few hours or overnight to allow the chia seeds to absorb the liquid and create a pudding-like consistency.
3. Top with ripe berries before serving.

Nutritional Value: Approximately 200 calories, 4g protein, 10g fat, 20g carbohydrates.

Preparation Time: 5 minutes + refrigeration time

13. RICE PORRIDGE WITH CINNAMON:

INGREDIENTS:

- 1/2 cup cooked white rice
- 1 cup almond milk
- 1/2 teaspoon cinnamon

INSTRUCTION

1. In a pot, combine cooked white rice and almond milk.
2. Cook over low heat, stirring occasionally, until the mixture thickens to a porridge consistency.
3. Stir in cinnamon and serve.

Nutritional Value: Approximately 200 calories, 2g protein, 5g fat, 35g carbohydrates.

Cooking Time: 15 minutes

14. NUT BUTTER BANANA WRAP:

INGREDIENTS:

- 1 whole-grain or corn tortilla
- 2 tablespoons almond butter or peanut butter
- 1 ripe banana

INSTRUCTION

1. Spread nut butter on the tortilla.
2. Place a ripe banana on one end and roll up the tortilla.

Nutritional Value: Approximately 300 calories, 5g protein, 10g fat, 45g carbohydrates.

Preparation Time: 5 minutes

15. LACTOSE-FREE YOGURT BOWL:

INGREDIENTS:

- 1 cup lactose-free yogurt
- 1/4 cup granola (low-fiber if needed)
- 1/4 cup sliced almonds

INSTRUCTION

1. In a bowl, layer lactose-free yogurt, granola, and sliced almonds.

Nutritional Value: Approximately 250 calories, 10g protein, 10g fat, 30g carbohydrates.

Preparation Time: 5 minutes

16. VEGGIE OMELETTE WRAP:

INGREDIENTS:

- 2 large eggs
- 1/4 cup diced bell peppers
- 1/4 cup diced tomatoes

- 1/4 cup diced cooked chicken or turkey

INSTRUCTION

1. In a bowl, whisk the eggs.
2. Heat a non-stick skillet over medium heat and pour in the eggs.
3. Sprinkle diced bell peppers, tomatoes, and cooked chicken on one half of the omelette.
4. Fold the other half over the filling and cook until set.
5. Serve the omelette wrapped in a soft tortilla.

Nutritional Value: Approximately 300 calories, 15g protein, 15g fat, 20g carbohydrates.

Cooking Time: 10 minutes

17. APPLE CINNAMON MUFFINS:

INGREDIENTS:

- 1 cup oat flour
- 1/2 teaspoon baking powder
- 1/2 teaspoon cinnamon
- 1/4 cup unsweetened applesauce
- 1/4 cup almond milk
- 1 tablespoon honey

INSTRUCTION

1. Preheat the oven to 350°F (175°C) and line a muffin tin with liners.
2. In a bowl, mix oat flour, baking powder, and cinnamon.
3. Add applesauce, almond milk, and honey. Mix until well combined.

4. Divide the batter into muffin cups and bake for about 15-20 minutes or until a toothpick comes out clean.

Nutritional Value: Approximately 150 calories, 3g protein, 2g fat, 30g carbohydrates.

Cooking Time: 20 minutes

18. QUINOA FRUIT SALAD:

INGREDIENTS:

- 1/2 cup cooked quinoa
- 1/2 cup ripe berries (blueberries, strawberries, raspberries)
- 1/2 cup diced ripe papaya

INSTRUCTION

1. In a bowl, combine cooked quinoa, ripe berries, and diced papaya.

Nutritional Value: Approximately 250 calories, 5g protein, 5g fat, 45g carbohydrates.

Preparation Time: 5 minutes

19. ALMOND MILK CHIA PUDDING:

INGREDIENTS:

- 2 tablespoons chia seeds
- 1/2 cup almond milk
- 1/4 teaspoon vanilla extract

INSTRUCTION

1. In a bowl, combine chia seeds, almond milk, and vanilla extract. Stir well.
2. Refrigerate for a few hours or overnight to allow the chia seeds to absorb the liquid and create a pudding-like consistency.
3. Serve as is or top with sliced fruits.

Nutritional Value: Approximately 150 calories, 3g protein, 8g fat, 15g carbohydrates.

Preparation Time: 5 minutes + refrigeration time

20. SOFT SCRAMBLED TOFU WITH VEGETABLES:

INGREDIENTS:

- 1/2 cup soft tofu, crumbled
- 1/4 cup diced bell peppers
- 1/4 cup diced zucchini
- 1/4 cup diced tomatoes
- Pinch of turmeric (for color)

INSTRUCTION

1. Heat a non-stick skillet over medium heat.
2. Add diced vegetables and sauté until slightly tender.
3. Add crumbled tofu and a pinch of turmeric for color. Cook until heated through.

Nutritional Value: Approximately 150 calories, 10g protein, 8g fat, 10g carbohydrates.

Cooking Time: 10 minutes

UC DIET LUNCH RECIPES

1. GRILLED CHICKEN AND RICE BOWL:

INGREDIENTS:

- 4 oz boneless, skinless chicken breast
- 1/2 cup cooked white rice
- 1/2 cup steamed carrots

INSTRUCTION

1. Season the chicken with salt and pepper.
2. Grill the chicken until fully cooked.
3. Serve over cooked white rice and steamed carrots.

Nutritional Value: Approximately 300 calories, 25g protein, 5g fat, 40g carbohydrates.

Cooking Time: 20 minutes

2. QUINOA AND VEGGIE STIR-FRY:

INGREDIENTS:

- 1/2 cup cooked quinoa
- 1/2 cup mixed vegetables (bell peppers, zucchini, carrots)
- 2 tablespoons low-sodium soy sauce

INSTRUCTION

1. Heat a non-stick skillet over medium heat.
2. Add mixed vegetables and stir-fry until slightly tender.
3. Add cooked quinoa and soy sauce. Stir-fry until heated through.

Nutritional Value: Approximately 250 calories, 8g protein, 5g fat, 40g carbohydrates.

Cooking Time: 15 minutes

3. BAKED SALMON WITH STEAMED BROCCOLI:

INGREDIENTS:

- 4 oz salmon fillet
- 1 cup steamed broccoli
- Lemon juice, for drizzling

INSTRUCTION

1. Preheat the oven to 375°F (190°C).
2. Place the salmon fillet on a baking sheet and bake until cooked through.
3. Serve with steamed broccoli and a drizzle of lemon juice.

Nutritional Value: Approximately 250 calories, 25g protein, 10g fat, 15g carbohydrates.

Cooking Time: 20 minutes

4. TOFU AND AVOCADO SALAD:

INGREDIENTS:

- 1 cup mixed salad greens
- 1/2 cup diced tofu
- 1/4 avocado, sliced
- 2 tablespoons balsamic vinaigrette

INSTRUCTION

1. Arrange salad greens on a plate.
2. Top with diced tofu and sliced avocado.
3. Drizzle with balsamic vinaigrette.

Nutritional value: Approximately 200 calories, 10g protein, 12g fat, 10g carbohydrates.

Preparation Time: 10 minutes

5. TURKEY AND RICE WRAP:

INGREDIENTS:

- 4 oz cooked turkey breast slices
- 1 whole-grain or corn tortilla
- 1/4 cup cooked white rice
- Lettuce and tomato slices, for filling

INSTRUCTION

1. Lay the tortilla flat and layer with turkey slices, cooked white rice, lettuce, and tomato slices.

2. Roll up the tortilla tightly to form a wrap.

Nutritional Value: Approximately 250 calories, 20g protein, 5g fat, 30g carbohydrates.

Preparation Time: 5 minutes

6. VEGGIE AND CHICKEN RICE BOWL:

INGREDIENTS:

- 4 oz cooked chicken breast, diced
- 1/2 cup cooked white rice
- 1/2 cup sautéed mixed vegetables (bell peppers, zucchini, carrots)

INSTRUCTION

1. Combine cooked chicken, cooked white rice, and sautéed mixed vegetables in a bowl.
2. Mix well and serve.

Nutritional Value: Approximately 300 calories, 25g protein, 5g fat, 40g carbohydrates.

Cooking Time: 20 minutes

7. LENTIL SOUP WITH TOASTED BREAD:

INGREDIENTS:

- 1 cup cooked lentils
- 1 cup low-sodium vegetable broth
- 1/2 cup diced carrots
- 1/4 cup diced celery
- 1 slice whole-grain bread

INSTRUCTION

1. In a pot, combine cooked lentils, vegetable broth, diced carrots, and diced celery.
2. Simmer until vegetables are tender.
3. Serve with a slice of toasted whole-grain bread.

Nutritional Value: Approximately 250 calories, 15g protein, 5g fat, 40g carbohydrates.

Cooking Time: 25 minutes

8. GREEK YOGURT AND BERRY PARFAIT:

INGREDIENTS:

- 1 cup lactose-free Greek yogurt
- 1/2 cup ripe berries (blueberries, strawberries, raspberries)
- 2 tablespoons chopped nuts (almonds, walnuts)

INSTRUCTION

1. In a glass, layer Greek yogurt, ripe berries, and chopped nuts.

Nutritional Value: Approximately 250 calories, 15g protein, 10g fat, 25g carbohydrates.

Preparation Time: 5 minutes

9. SPINACH AND FETA OMELETTE:

INGREDIENTS:

- 2 large eggs
- 1/2 cup fresh spinach, chopped
- 1/4 cup crumbled feta cheese

INSTRUCTION

1. In a bowl, whisk the eggs.
2. Heat a non-stick skillet over medium heat and pour in the eggs.
3. Sprinkle chopped spinach and crumbled feta cheese on one half of the omelette.
4. Fold the other half over the filling and cook until set.

Nutritional Value: Approximately 250 calories, 20g protein, 15g fat, 5g carbohydrates.

Cooking Time: 10 minutes

10. VEGGIE AND HUMMUS WRAP:

INGREDIENTS:

- 1 whole-grain or corn tortilla
- 2 tablespoons hummus
- Sliced cucumber, bell peppers, and carrots, for filling

INSTRUCTION

1. Spread hummus evenly on the tortilla.
2. Place sliced cucumber, bell peppers, and carrots on top of the hummus.
3. Roll up the tortilla tightly to form a wrap.

Nutritional Value: Approximately 200 calories, 5g protein, 8g fat, 30g carbohydrates.

Preparation Time: 5 minutes

11. RICE NOODLE SALAD WITH CHICKEN:

INGREDIENTS:

- 4 oz cooked chicken breast, shredded
- 1 cup cooked rice noodles
- 1/2 cup shredded carrots
- 1/4 cup sliced cucumber
- 2 tablespoons low-sodium soy sauce

INSTRUCTION

1. In a bowl, combine shredded chicken, cooked rice noodles, shredded carrots, and sliced cucumber.
2. Drizzle with low-sodium soy sauce and toss to combine.

Nutritional Value: Approximately 300 calories, 20g protein, 5g fat, 45g carbohydrates.

Preparation Time: 15 minutes

12. MIXED GREENS AND QUINOA SALAD:

INGREDIENTS:

- 1 cup mixed salad greens
- 1/2 cup cooked quinoa
- 1/4 cup diced cucumber
- 1/4 cup diced bell peppers
- 2 tablespoons olive oil and vinegar dressing

INSTRUCTION

1. In a bowl, combine mixed salad greens, cooked quinoa, diced cucumber, and diced bell peppers.
2. Drizzle with olive oil and vinegar dressing.

Nutritional Value: Approximately 250 calories, 8g protein, 10g fat, 30g carbohydrates.

Preparation Time: 10 minutes

13. GRILLED VEGGIE WRAP:

INGREDIENTS:

- 1 whole-grain or corn tortilla
- 1/4 cup hummus
- Grilled vegetables (bell peppers, zucchini, eggplant), for filling

INSTRUCTION

1. Spread hummus evenly on the tortilla.
2. Place grilled vegetables on top of the hummus.
3. Roll up the tortilla tightly to form a wrap.

Nutritional Value: Approximately 200 calories, 4g protein, 6g fat, 30g carbohydrates.

Preparation Time: 10 minutes

14. TURKEY AND AVOCADO LETTUCE WRAPS:

INGREDIENTS:

- 4 oz cooked turkey breast slices
- Large lettuce leaves (such as Romaine)
- 1/4 avocado, sliced
- Sliced tomatoes, for filling

- INSTRUCTION

1. Lay lettuce leaves flat and layer with turkey slices, avocado slices, and sliced tomatoes.
2. Roll up the lettuce leaves to form wraps.

Nutritional Value: Approximately 200 calories, 15g protein, 6g fat, 20g carbohydrates.

Preparation Time: 10 minutes

15. BAKED SWEET POTATO WITH BLACK BEANS:

INGREDIENTS:

- 1 medium sweet potato
- 1/2 cup cooked black beans
- Salsa or diced tomatoes, for topping

INSTRUCTION

1. Preheat the oven to 400°F (200°C).
2. Pierce the sweet potato with a fork and bake until tender.
3. Cut open the sweet potato and top with cooked black beans and salsa or diced tomatoes.

Nutritional Value: Approximately 250 calories, 10g protein, 1g fat, 50g carbohydrates.

Cooking Time 40 minutes

16. HUMMUS AND VEGGIE WRAP:

INGREDIENTS:

- 1 whole-grain or corn tortilla
- 1/4 cup hummus
- Sliced bell peppers, cucumber, and carrots, for filling

INSTRUCTION

1. Spread hummus evenly on the tortilla.
2. Place sliced bell peppers, cucumber, and carrots on top of the hummus.
3. Roll up the tortilla tightly to form a wrap.

Nutritional Value: Approximately 200 calories, 4g protein, 6g fat, 30g carbohydrates.

Preparation Time: 10 minutes

17. GRILLED TOFU AND VEGGIE SKEWERS:

INGREDIENTS:

- 4 oz firm tofu, cubed
- Assorted vegetables (bell peppers, zucchini, cherry tomatoes), cut into chunks
- Olive oil, for brushing

INSTRUCTION

1. Preheat the grill or grill pan.
2. Thread tofu cubes and vegetable chunks onto skewers.
3. Brush with olive oil and grill until vegetables are tender and tofu is lightly browned.

Nutritional Value: Approximately 200 calories, 10g protein, 8g fat, 20g carbohydrates.

Cooking Time: 15 minutes

18. EGG SALAD LETTUCE WRAPS:

INGREDIENTS:

- 2 hard-boiled eggs, chopped
- 1 tablespoon mayonnaise (or dairy-free alternative)
- Lettuce leaves (such as butter lettuce or Romaine)

INSTRUCTION

1. In a bowl, mix chopped hard-boiled eggs and mayonnaise.
2. Spoon the egg salad onto lettuce leaves and wrap them up.

Nutritional Value: Approximately 200 calories, 10g protein, 15g fat, 5g carbohydrates.

Preparation Time: 15 minutes

19. QUINOA AND BLACK BEAN BOWL:

INGREDIENTS:

- 1/2 cup cooked quinoa
- 1/2 cup cooked black beans
- 1/4 cup diced tomatoes
- 1/4 cup diced bell peppers
- 2 tablespoons chopped fresh cilantro

INSTRUCTION

1. In a bowl, combine cooked quinoa, black beans, diced tomatoes, diced bell peppers, and chopped cilantro.

Nutritional Value: Approximately 250 calories, 10g protein, 3g fat, 45g carbohydrates.

Preparation Time: 10 minutes

:

20. CREAMY TOMATO SOUP WITH RICE CAKES:

INGREDIENTS:

- 1 cup low-sodium tomato soup (lactose-free if needed)
- 2 rice cakes
- Fresh basil leaves, for garnish

INSTRUCTION

1. Heat the tomato soup in a pot until warmed through.
2. Serve with rice cakes on the side and garnish with fresh basil leaves.

Nutritional Value: Approximately 150 calories, 2g protein, 1g fat, 30g carbohydrates.

Cooking Time: 10 minutes

UC DIET DINNER RECIPES

1. BAKED SALMON WITH QUINOA AND STEAMED ASPARAGUS:

INGREDIENTS:

- 4 oz salmon fillet
- 1/2 cup cooked quinoa
- 1 cup steamed asparagus

INSTRUCTION

1. Preheat the oven to 375°F (190°C).
2. Place the salmon fillet on a baking sheet and bake until cooked through.
3. Serve with cooked quinoa and steamed asparagus.

Nutritional Value: Approximately 300 calories, 25g protein, 10g fat, 25g carbohydrates.

Cooking Time: 20 minutes

2. GRILLED CHICKEN WITH MASHED POTATOES AND GREEN BEANS:

INGREDIENTS:

- 4 oz boneless, skinless chicken breast
- 1/2 cup mashed potatoes (made with lactose-free milk)
- 1 cup steamed green beans

INSTRUCTION

1. Season the chicken with salt and pepper.
2. Grill the chicken until fully cooked.
3. Serve with mashed potatoes and steamed green beans.

Nutritional Value: Approximately 300 calories, 25g protein, 5g fat, 40g carbohydrates.

Cooking Time: 25 minutes

3. LENTIL AND VEGETABLE STIR-FRY:

INGREDIENTS:

- 1/2 cup cooked lentils
- 1 cup mixed vegetables (bell peppers, zucchini, carrots)
- 2 tablespoons low-sodium soy sauce

INSTRUCTION

1. Heat a non-stick skillet over medium heat.
2. Add mixed vegetables and stir-fry until slightly tender.
3. Add cooked lentils and soy sauce. Stir-fry until heated through.

Nutritional Value: Approximately 250 calories, 10g protein, 2g fat, 45g carbohydrates.

Cooking Time: 15 minutes

4. QUINOA AND BLACK BEAN STUFFED BELL PEPPERS:

INGREDIENTS:

- 2 bell peppers, halved and seeds removed
- 1 cup cooked quinoa
- 1/2 cup cooked black beans
- 1/4 cup diced tomatoes
- 2 tablespoons shredded dairy-free cheese (optional)

INSTRUCTION

1. Preheat the oven to 375°F (190°C).
2. In a bowl, combine cooked quinoa, black beans, and diced tomatoes.
4. Stuff the bell pepper halves with the quinoa mixture.

5. Place the stuffed peppers on a baking sheet, cover with foil, and bake until the peppers are tender.

6. If using, sprinkle shredded dairy-free cheese on top and bake until melted.

Nutritional Value: Approximately 300 calories, 10g protein, 5g fat, 50g carbohydrates.

Cooking Time: 30 minutes

5. VEGETABLE AND TOFU STIR-FRY WITH RICE:

INGREDIENTS:

- 1/2 cup cooked brown rice
- 1/2 cup mixed vegetables (bell peppers, broccoli, carrots)
- 4 oz firm tofu, cubed
- 2 tablespoons low-sodium stir-fry sauce

INSTRUCTION

1. Heat a non-stick skillet over medium heat.
2. Add mixed vegetables and stir-fry until slightly tender.
3. Push the vegetables to the side of the skillet and add tofu cubes. Cook until lightly browned.
4. Combine vegetables, tofu, and cooked brown rice in the skillet.
5. Drizzle with low-sodium stir-fry sauce and stir-fry until heated through.

Nutritional Value: Approximately 300 calories, 15g protein, 5g fat, 50g carbohydrates.

Cooking Time: 20 minutes

6. TOMATO BASIL CHICKEN SOUP:

INGREDIENTS:

- 4 oz cooked chicken breast, shredded
- 1 cup low-sodium chicken broth
- 1/2 cup diced tomatoes
- 1/4 cup cooked rice

INSTRUCTION

1. In a pot, combine shredded chicken, chicken broth, diced tomatoes, and cooked rice.
2. Simmer until heated through.
3. Serve with fresh basil leaves as garnish.

Nutritional Value: Approximately 250 calories, 20g protein, 2g fat, 35g carbohydrates.

Cooking Time: 15 minutes

7. SPINACH AND CHICKPEA SALAD WITH GRILLED CHICKEN:

INGREDIENTS:

- 4 oz grilled chicken breast, sliced
- 2 cups fresh spinach
- 1/2 cup cooked chickpeas
- 1/4 cup diced cucumber
- 1/4 cup diced red onion
- 2 tablespoons balsamic vinaigrette

INSTRUCTION

1. In a bowl, combine fresh spinach, cooked chickpeas, diced cucumber, and diced red onion.
2. Top with sliced grilled chicken.
3. Drizzle with balsamic vinaigrette.

Nutritional Value: Approximately 300 calories, 25g protein, 8g fat, 30g carbohydrates.

Preparation Time: 15 minutes

8. VEGETABLE AND RICE NOODLE STIR-FRY:

INGREDIENTS:

- 1/2 cup cooked rice noodles
- 1/2 cup mixed vegetables (bell peppers, broccoli, carrots)
- 2 tablespoons low-sodium soy sauce
- 1 tablespoon sesame oil

INSTRUCTION

1. Cook rice noodles according to package instructions.
2. Heat sesame oil in a pan over medium heat.
3. Add mixed vegetables and stir-fry until slightly tender.

4. Add cooked rice noodles and drizzle with low-sodium soy sauce. Stir-fry until heated through.

Nutritional Value: Approximately 250 calories, 5g protein, 8g fat, 40g carbohydrates.

Cooking Time: 15 minutes

9. STUFFED ACORN SqUASH WITH QUINOA AND KALE:

INGREDIENTS:

- 1 acorn squash, halved and seeds removed
- 1/2 cup cooked quinoa
- 1 cup chopped kale
- 1/4 cup chopped walnuts

INSTRUCTION

1. Preheat the oven to 375°F (190°C).
2. Place the acorn squash halves on a baking sheet and bake until tender.

3. In a bowl, combine cooked quinoa, chopped kale, and chopped walnuts.

4. Fill the acorn squash halves with the quinoa mixture.

5. Return to the oven and bake for a few more minutes until heated through.

Nutritional Value: Approximately 300 calories, 8g protein, 10g fat, 45g carbohydrates.

Cooking Time: 40 minutes

10. BAKED CHICKEN AND SWEET POTATO FRIES:

INGREDIENTS:

- 4 oz boneless, skinless chicken breast
- 1 medium sweet potato, cut into fries
- 1 tablespoon olive oil
- Dash of paprika and garlic powder

INSTRUCTION

1. Preheat the oven to 400°F (200°C).

2. Toss sweet potato fries with olive oil, paprika, and garlic powder.

3. Place chicken breast and sweet potato fries on a baking sheet.

4. Bake until the chicken is cooked through and the sweet potato fries are crispy.

Nutritional Value: Approximately 300 calories, 25g protein, 8g fat, 30g carbohydrates.

Cooking Time: 30 minutes

11. MEDITERRANEAN GRILLED VEGGIE AND QUINOA SALAD:

INGREDIENTS:

- 1/2 cup cooked quinoa
- Grilled vegetables (eggplant, zucchini, red onion, bell peppers)

- 1/4 cup chopped fresh parsley
- 2 tablespoons lemon juice

INSTRUCTION

1. Combine cooked quinoa and grilled vegetables in a bowl.
2. Toss with chopped fresh parsley and lemon juice.

Nutritional Value: Approximately 250 calories, 5g protein, 8g fat, 40g carbohydrates.

Preparation Time: 20 minutes

12. TOFU STIR-FRY WITH BROCCOLI AND CASHEWS:

INGREDIENTS:

- 4 oz firm tofu, cubed
- 1 cup steamed broccoli florets
- 2 tablespoons low-sodium stir-fry sauce

- 2 tablespoons chopped cashews

INSTRUCTION

1. Heat a non-stick skillet over medium heat.
2. Add cubed tofu and stir-fry until lightly browned.
3. Add steamed broccoli and stir-fry sauce. Stir-fry until heated through.
4. Sprinkle chopped cashews on top before serving.

Nutritional Value: Approximately 300 calories, 15g protein, 10g fat, 25g carbohydrates.

Cooking Time: 15 minutes

13. BAKED COD WITH ROASTED VEGETABLES:

INGREDIENTS:

- 4 oz cod fillet
- Assorted roasted vegetables (carrots, bell peppers, zucchini)
- 1 tablespoon olive oil

INSTRUCTION

1. Preheat the oven to 375°F (190°C).
2. Place the cod fillet on a baking sheet and drizzle with olive oil.
3. Bake until the cod is cooked through.
4. Serve with assorted roasted vegetables.

Nutritional Value: Approximately 250 calories, 20g protein, 8g fat, 25g carbohydrates.

Cooking Time: 20 minutes

14. SPINACH AND TOMATO OMELETTE:

INGREDIENTS:

- 3 large eggs
- 1/2 cup fresh spinach, chopped
- 1/4 cup diced tomatoes
- 2 tablespoons shredded dairy-free cheese (optional)

INSTRUCTION

1. In a bowl, whisk the eggs.
2. Heat a non-stick skillet over medium heat and pour in the eggs.
3. Sprinkle chopped spinach, diced tomatoes, and shredded dairy-free cheese on one half of the omelette.
4. Fold the other half over the filling and cook until set.

Nutritional Value: Approximately 250 calories, 15g protein, 15g fat, 5g carbohydrates.

Cooking Time: 10 minutes

15. VEGGIE BURGER WITH SWEET POTATO FRIES:

INGREDIENTS:

- 1 veggie burger patty (lactose-free if needed)
- 1 whole-grain bun
- Baked sweet potato fries
- Lettuce, tomato, and onion slices, for topping

INSTRUCTION

2. Cook the veggie burger patty according to package instructions.
3. Assemble the burger by placing the patty on the whole-grain bun.

4. Top with lettuce, tomato, and onion slices.

5. Serve with a side of baked sweet potato fries.

Nutritional Value: Approximately 300 calories, 10g protein, 8g fat, 50g carbohydrates.

Cooking Time: 20 minutes

16. RICE AND BEAN BOWL WITH SAUTÉED SPINACH:

INGREDIENTS:

- 1/2 cup cooked brown rice
- 1/2 cup cooked black beans
- 1 cup sautéed spinach
- 1 tablespoon olive oil

INSTRUCTION

1. Heat olive oil in a pan over medium heat.

6. Add sautéed spinach and cook until wilted.

7. Combine cooked brown rice and black beans in a bowl.
8. Serve with sautéed spinach on top.

Nutritional Value: Approximately 250 calories, 10g protein, 8g fat, 40g carbohydrates.

Cooking Time: 15 minutes

17. TURKEY AND VEGETABLE SKILLET:

INGREDIENTS:

- 4 oz cooked ground turkey
- 1 cup mixed vegetables (bell peppers, zucchini, carrots)
- 1/4 cup low-sodium tomato sauce
- 1/2 teaspoon Italian seasoning

INSTRUCTION

1. Heat a skillet over medium heat.

2. Add cooked ground turkey and mixed vegetables. Cook until vegetables are tender.

3. Stir in low-sodium tomato sauce and Italian seasoning. Heat through.

Nutritional Value: Approximately 250 calories, 20g protein, 8g fat, 25g carbohydrates.

Cooking Time: 15 minutes

18. EGGPLANT AND TOMATO PASTA:

INGREDIENTS:

- 1 cup cooked gluten-free pasta (lactose-free if needed)
- 1 cup diced eggplant
- 1/2 cup diced tomatoes
- 2 tablespoons olive oil
- Fresh basil leaves, for garnish

INSTRUCTION

1. Heat olive oil in a pan over medium heat.

4. Add diced eggplant and cook until tender.

5. Stir in diced tomatoes and cooked pasta. Heat through.

6. Garnish with fresh basil leaves before serving.

Nutritional Value: Approximately 300 calories, 5g protein, 10g fat, 45g carbohydrates.

Cooking Time: 20 minutes

19. CHICKEN AND VEGETABLE SKEWERS WITH QUINOA:

INGREDIENTS:

- 4 oz grilled chicken breast, cubed
- Assorted vegetables (bell peppers, onions, zucchini), cut into chunks
- 1/2 cup cooked quinoa

- 2 tablespoons lemon juice

INSTRUCTION

1. Thread chicken cubes and vegetable chunks onto skewers.
2. Grill until the chicken is cooked through and vegetables are tender.
3. Serve with cooked quinoa and drizzle with lemon juice.

Nutritional Value: Approximately 300 calories, 25g protein, 5g fat, 40g carbohydrates.

Cooking Time: 20 minutes

20. ZUCCHINI NOODLES WITH PESTO AND CHERRY TOMATOES:

INGREDIENTS:

- 2 medium zucchinis, spiralized into noodles
- 2 tablespoons dairy-free pesto
- 1/2 cup halved cherry tomatoes

- 1 tablespoon pine nuts (optional)

INSTRUCTION

1. In a pan, sauté zucchini noodles until tender.
2. Toss with dairy-free pesto and halved cherry tomatoes.
3. If using, sprinkle pine nuts on top before serving.

Nutritional Value: Approximately 250 calories, 5g protein, 20g fat, 15g carbohydrates.

Cooking Time: 15 minutes

CONCLUSION

This comprehensive Ulcerative Colitis Disease Cookbook serves as a valuable resource for individuals seeking to manage their condition through a balanced and flavorful dietary approach. By understanding the disease types, causes, symptoms, and complications associated with ulcerative colitis, you've gained the necessary knowledge to make informed choices about your diet. The carefully curated recipes provided here offer a diverse array of flavorful options that not only cater to your health needs but also satisfy your taste buds. From nutrient-packed breakfasts to satisfying lunches and dinners, this cookbook empowers you with the tools to create meals that support your well-being without compromising on taste. By embracing an ulcerative colitis-friendly diet, you're taking proactive steps towards alleviating symptoms and promoting gut health. The ingredients and preparation methods offered are not just recipes, but gateways to managing your condition and achieving optimum health.

Remember, embarking on this dietary journey requires patience and dedication. While each individual's experience with ulcerative colitis may differ, the core principles of this cookbook remain steadfast: embracing whole foods, avoiding triggers, and prioritizing nutrient-rich ingredients. Your health and well-being are worth the investment, and by adopting and adapting these recipes, you are taking control of your journey towards a balanced and fulfilling life. So, whether you're just starting out or looking to expand your culinary horizons, let this cookbook be your guide. Every meal is an opportunity to nurture your body and find joy in the process. By making choices that honor your health, you're not only nourishing your physical being but also cultivating resilience and a profound sense of well-being. So, go ahead, savor the flavors, and enjoy the positive impact of a well-crafted diet tailored to your unique needs.

Your journey to better health starts in your kitchen – it's time to take that empowering step forward.

Printed in Great Britain
by Amazon